Lose 16 Pounds In 12-Days On A Smoothie Cleanse Diet: Rapidly Lose Weight, Fight Cancerous Diseases, And Look Younger Whilst Drinking A Delicious Green Smoothie

ISBN: 9798651256174
Ebook ASIN: B089NJXMD6

Acknowledgement

I want to thank you and congratulate you for downloading the book, **"Lose 16 Pounds in 12-Days On A Smoothie Cleanse Diet"**.

If you interested in learning the latest scientific breakthroughs in fat loss? You are not alone! Millions for people all over the world are trying to lose weight and do so in a safe and effective manner.

What I have done is put together 3 totally *FREE e-books* to get you started on the road to success. These reports won't be up forever, so get them before they are taken down.

It's my simple way of saying thank you for downloading this book.

CLICK HERE TO GET INSTANCE ACCESS
or
https://stephaniequinones6.wixsite.com/freereports

Download 3 of the BEST E-books ABSOLUTELY FREE that will help you lose weight, melt off fat, and get in great shape!

Report #1: Top Delicious Fruits for Weight Loss

Report #2: 10 Easiest Fat-Trimming Workouts for Weight Loss

Report #3: Top 4 Tips for Getting Rid of Belly Fat

Other Books by Stephanie Quiñones

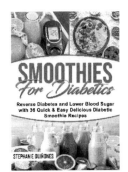

<u>**Smoothies for Diabetics: Reverse Diabetes and Lower Blood Sugar with 36 Quick & Easy Delicious Diabetic Smoothie Recipes**</u>

****

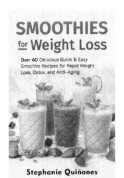

<u>**Smoothies for Weight Loss: Over 60 Delicious Quick & Easy Smoothie Recipes for Rapid Weight Loss, Detox, and Anti-Aging**</u>

TABLE OF CONTENT

INTRODUCTION

CHAPTER 1: THE GREEN SMOOTHIE CLEANSE DIET

CHAPTER 2: THE 12-DAY GREEN SMOOTHIE MEAL
REPLACEMENT PLAN
    WEEK ONE
    WEEK TWO

CHAPTER 3: MORE GREEN SMOOTHIE RECIPES

CHAPTER 4: HEALTHY SNACKING AND EXERCISING

CHAPTER 5: TRACK YOUR PROGRESS AND SEE RESULTS
    WEEK ONE GREEN SMOOTHIE MEAL PLAN
    WEEK TWO OF GREEN SMOOTHIE DIET
    CONTINUE THE PLAN AFTER THE 12 DAYS!

CONCLUSION

THANK YOU

ABOUT AUTHOR

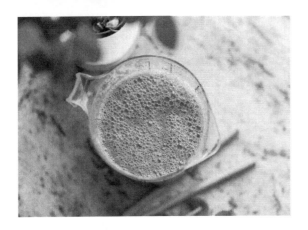

INTRODUCTION

Gaining weight sucks. For one, all the old clothes that you love don't seem to fit anymore, and you have to suck your belly in before you can fit in those tight jeans, and I know you will agree with me when I say that it can be pure torture. Once you have that excess weight, it sometimes feels like your dresses do not fit you as much as they used to, and it is sad to put them aside because they are now two or more sizes smaller than you. Everyone wants to look their best, and while some find comfort in working their asses off at the gym to get the body that they want, most of us would prefer to find an easy way around it without stressing ourselves with all the workouts.

If you are losing to lose weight without having to do lots of workouts, the next best thing to consider is food as what you put in your body can either make or break your weight loss goals. Even if you work out day and night, as long as what you eat isn't healthy, it will take a long time for you to see the results; longer than you ever expected. So, while putting in as much work as you can, try to focus on your food and what better way to do so than smoothies. Filled with all sorts of deliciousness, smoothies are the best way to get your day started and shed that extra weight without breaking a muscle, and in this book, we will show you just how much smoothies can make a difference in your weight loss goals.

In this book, we will be discussing green smoothies and the best ingredients you can use to make them. A lot of people don't like green smoothies because a lot of them do not have the best taste, but after finding a way around it, green smoothies are my new favorite, and I can show you the surprising ingredient that makes it all worthwhile. Sit back and enjoy a good read.

CHAPTER 1

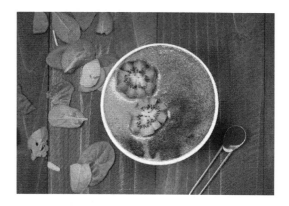

THE GREEN SMOOTHIE CLEANSE DIET

If you are a fan of reading lifestyle blogs or watching the Instagram stories of some of your favorite celebrities, you will realize that most of them swear by detox and cleansing as the way they maintain their fit bodies. In the last few years, there has been a tremendous increase in people with obesity and other fat-related issues that the need for rapid weight loss programs and tips has become so sought after. The main essence of cleansing is to rid your body of the toxins that make you gain weight and prevent weight loss by cutting out all the foods that do your body no good. Cleansing is a chance for your body to reset and get back to the way it once was without the junks and unhealthy foods standing in your way. You might say, "But the body has its way of clearing toxins, so why do I still need to do a body cleanse?" Yes, the body does indeed have its way of removing toxins, which is through the liver, sweat, urine, and feces, but the body still needs the help which cleansing provides to neutralize toxins without putting a strain on the organs responsible for doing so. What makes a body cleanse so special?

A cleanse involves the consumption of liquids and the removal of unhealthy food, some of which you are already attached to. Many of us cannot see ourselves spending the day without a bottle of coke or having a hamburger, and it feels like the world does not make sense anymore once we start cutting some of those foods out of our diet. A cleanse does not completely stop your cravings but instead gives you control in such a way that you might be thinking about them, but you will have the power to resist eating them. The liquids you take during a cleanse fill you up and help to subdue your cravings. The first few days of the cleanse might feel like hell because you had removes foods that you cherish, but as you stick to the plan and keep your mind away from those unhealthy foods, you would find it easier to continue the cleanse and by the time you are done, your addiction to such unhealthy food will be a thing of the past. Some of the foods we eat are made up of substances that do the body no good in the long-run, and some of the chemicals in the foods have started affecting the body, which has resulted in the weight gain. Since a cleanse removes processed foods and refined sugars from your diet, it helps to support the body's digestive process and reduce bloating and constipation. Majority of the foods and supplements taken during a cleanse are easy to digest, and they help the body remove the toxins that put a strain on the body.

Since your liver is not working overtime to break down the food you eat, that leaves your body with a lot of energy to carry out daily functions. So, instead of feeling sluggish and tired before the day has started, you will find yourself bursting with energy, leaving you refreshed by the end of the day. According to a German research study, when we are tired or stressed out, the body releases a hormone called cortisol, which reduces the liver function. When you do a cleanse, it helps you manage your stress, and the cortisol levels in the body are reduced by managing your stress. Eating processed foods and refined sugars contributes greatly to fatigue, and by eliminating it from your diet, you are giving your liver a fresh start. Also, the toxins in your body can hurt your sleep patterns and leave you feeling sluggish and tired throughout the day. Cleansing helps you feel renewed and rejuvenated anytime you start your day.

There are different types of cleanses, but since the green smoothie diet is our major focus, let's get into it. Green smoothies are a blended combination of leafy greens with fruits, vegetables, and a little bit of healthy fat. You can choose to make your green smoothies with anything you love, but the ingredients commonly used are kale, Swiss chard, mint, collard greens, and parsley, plus, you can choose to use fresh fruits or frozen fruits for your smoothie. As if being delicious was not enough, green smoothies help to lower cholesterol and glucose levels because of its high fiber content. Because of its fiber content, green smoothies help to keep you fuller and increase your body's ability to burn fat. Eating fruits and vegetables can sometimes get tiring, and you might not be able to eat as much as you would like. By taking green smoothies, you have all the ingredients you need in one glass. Drinking leafy greens alone might not encourage you to keep up with your green smoothie diet, but with the addition of fruits in it, you won't even feel any of the greens you put in it. All the nutrients you get from green smoothies, helps to strengthen your immune system thereby increasing your body's ability to defend itself against harmful diseases. Plus, green smoothies also provide your body with lots of antioxidants so not only are you equipping your body with the equipment it needs to fight against diseases, you are also giving it key nutrients that will help boost your health and fitness. Have you ever thought of replacing your early morning coffee with a glass of smoothie every morning? If you have not, now might be a good time to reconsider as green smoothies helps to increase your focus and mental wellbeing without any of the side effects of coffee. That is, you can stay in great mental shape throughout the day without feeling fatigued, which is what happens when your coffee has started wearing off.

There are a lot of creams, masks, and drugs out there, all promising to give you the clear skin and good hair that you have always wanted; meanwhile, all you need is to incorporate green smoothies to your diet. Drinking green smoothies helps to give you a healthy glow and can make your nails, hair, and skin look healthier and stronger. With all the nutrients that green smoothies provide, it is no surprise that going on a smoothie diet can help reduce the risk of developing diseases such as diabetes, obesity, cancer, cardiovascular disease, and other age-related conditions. When you combine green smoothies with a healthy diet, it can also help reduce your chances of stroke, Lupus, Parkinson's disease, Fibromyalgia, and other health conditions.

The first three days of your green smoothie diet will be anything but easy as your body is trying to adjust itself to the new normal. Since your body is used to receiving a large number of calories from the foods you eat, you will now have to make do with the small number of calories you get from your smoothies. During the first three days, try not to succumb to your body's need for whole foods and junks, and if you stick to it, your cravings will start to lessen. If early morning coffee is a part of your everyday routine, starting this green smoothie diet is a time to let your body rest. Coffee is acidic and has caffeine, which gives your body a rush, and as a result of this, it prevents the body from being in an alkaline state. Avoiding anything with caffeine is extremely important when starting the diet, but if you really feel the need to take coffee, try taking green tea instead but a small amount of it. As you start your 12-day green smoothie diet, you are not allowed to just eat anything. As has been mentioned earlier, you need to stay away from foods like sugar, bread, alcohol, soy, dairy milk, corn, gluten, wheat, red meat, diet soda (or any type of soda), coffee (or any product with caffeine), donuts, pasta, etc. If you are really missing the foods you used to eat, you can try incorporating some healthy snacks into your diet such as apple celery, carrots, unsweetened peanut butter, cucumbers, hard-boiled eggs, deviled eggs, and some unsalted nuts and seeds. During your diet, do not forget to drink at least eight glasses of water every day, and if you feel water alone is not your style, try mixing things up by drinking some herbal teas in place of water once in a while. Apart from taking lots of water and snacks, exercising would also be beneficial during this diet, and by exercise, I do not mean the rigorous backbreaking routines that we do at the gym. Do some stretches and remember not to stress yourself out during those exercises.

On the 12th and final day of your diet, pat yourself on the back for seeing it through and sticking with your goals because those 12 days had most likely been torture for you. After achieving your weight loss goals, the next most important step is keeping the weight off. If you revert to your old eating pattern which resulted in you gaining weight in the first place, all your hard work would be for nothing as the weight would come back, and you would have to go through the process over again. After your green smoothie diet, do not just jump back into eating whole foods, and eating salads would be a good way to start your return back to healthy eating. For the first two to three days after your diet, have a green smoothie every morning and have some sautéed vegetables for lunch and dinner. The goal here is to get used to eating light foods so that your body won't feel bloated and nausea won't set in. You can also try replacing carbs with fats and protein. By eating healthier fats and proteins in place of carbs, you are curbing your hunger and losing weight (or maintaining your weight) since you are eating lesser calories. Try replacing your high carb meals with protein-rich meals like chicken, eggs, salmon, sardines, lean beef, beans, milk, cheese, yogurt, and the likes. When it comes to eating fats, it is best to eat foods with unsaturated fats as they are healthy and an important aspect of a healthy diet, foods with unsaturated fat include avocados, olives or olive oil, peanut butter, sunflower, canola, fatty fish like salmon and mackerel, and nuts and seeds like almonds, chia seeds, peanuts, cashews, and sesame seeds.

CHAPTER 2

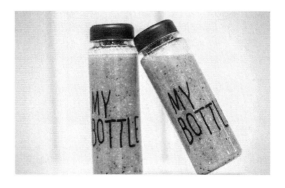

THE 12-DAY GREEN SMOOTHIE MEAL REPLACEMENT PLAN

It is the moment we have all been waiting for. It is time to motivate yourself with a lot of pep talk because your 12-day green smoothie diet is about to start. On the day before you start your new meal plan, enjoy your favorite meal because you won't be touching it anytime soon. Remember to stick to the plan and try as much as you can to see it through. When it seems like you cannot go further anymore, try to remind yourself why you started the diet in the first place and what your weight goals are for the rest of the diet. You had faced other challenges before and conquered them, and this is not the time for you to give up and quit. Without much ado, let us get into it.

YOUR SHOPPING LIST

If you haven't already gotten the fruits and vegetables you are going to use, or do not know what to get for the diet, do not worry I have got your back.

It is time to go shopping for your 12-day green smoothie meal plan. Grab your shopping cart and get (the quantity you want is left to you). When shopping, get enough fruits and vegetables to last you for the first week and when you are done with the first seven days, go back and get some more for the second week. These are the ingredients you should get for the first week:

- Apples
- Grapes
- Frozen Peaches
- Bananas

- Spinach
- Swiss Chard
- Coconut Milk and oil
- Water
- Pear
- Avocados
- Pineapples
- Chia seeds
- Flax seeds
- Turmeric powder
- Kale
- Stevia (to sweeten)
- Berries of different kinds like blueberries, strawberries etc.
- Spring mix greens
- Unsweetened peanut butter and nuts to snack on
- Plant based protein powder (optional)
- Greek yoghurt
- Almond milk

If you are new to the green smoothie diet, it is best that you do not rush into it as you might find yourself rushing out before the end of the meal plan. Gently ease into it by taking two glasses of smoothie for breakfast and lunch and having a healthy meal for dinner. A salad, sautéed vegetables and grilled chicken are excellent choices. After the first two to three days, try taking green smoothies three times a day and when you feel hungry, you can try eating a healthy snack to compliment the smoothies. Your green smoothies should be a blend of water, fruits and vegetables and as much as you can, avoid going for starchy vegetables like carrots, beets, zucchini and other non-leafy vegetables. When blending your ingredients, make sure you do it in stages in order to avoid chunky leafy vegetables in your smoothie and try to follow the 60/40 formula when making your smoothie. If this is your first green smoothie diet, you do not want to throw just anything into the blender as it might come out nasty and dissuade you from going through with the diet. Take out some measuring cups and make sure that 60% of your ingredients are fruits while the other 40% is leafy vegetables.

After shopping, it is time to bring out your scale and take measurements of yourself so that you can keep track of your progress during the diet. Take a photo of your body as well so that you will be able to see the physical changes that your body undergoes during the diet. That way, you can monitor your total progress.

WEEK ONE

- [ ] **Breakfast Green Smoothie:** This is the first smoothie of the day and it is going to be the backbone on which the rest of your day operates. To make your breakfast smoothie you will need:

- [ ] 1 banana
- [ ] ½ of an apple
- [ ] 2 tablespoons of chia seeds (if you are not a newbie, you can use it according to your discretion)
- [ ] 1-2 cups of water
- [ ] 1-2 cups of pineapple
- [ ] 2 cups of spinach or kale (use the one available)

- [ ] **Nutritional Facts:**

Calories: 202kcal
Cholesterol: 20mg
Total fats: 8g
Sugar: 35g
Fiber: 2g
Protein: 7g

- [ ] **Lunch Green Smoothie:** How are you feeling? It is time for your lunch smoothie. For this you will need:

- [ ] 6oz of Greek yoghurt
- [ ] Coconut milk
- [ ] 1 ripe or frozen banana (depending on what you have)
- [ ] 2-4 cups of Spinach or Kale
- [ ] Water

- [ ] **Nutritional Facts:**

Calories: 250kcal
Cholesterol: 0mg
Total fats: 9g
Sugar: 35g
Fiber: 2g
Protein: 5g

If you are using a high powered blender, place all the ingredients in the blender and blend it slowly while adding water at regular intervals to prevent chunky vegetables. Blend for 5 minutes and your lunch smoothie is ready. If you have kids and you want them to drink the smoothie with you, try adding blueberries in it so that the color would change and they won't know that they are drinking a smoothie with veggies in it.

- [ ] **Dinner green smoothie:** As I mentioned earlier, the first three days of the diet is going to be a struggle and if you feel like you need some food in your system, try eating something light like a salad or sautéed vegetables. If you feel you are good to go, you will need these ingredients for your dinner smoothie:

- [ ] Water
- [ ] Protein powder (optional)
- [ ] 2 handfuls of spinach
- [ ] Berries (either blueberries or strawberries)
- [ ] Chia seeds
- [ ] 1 handful of Swiss chard

- [ ] **Nutritional Facts:**

Calories: 184kcal
Cholesterol: 10mg
Total fats: 1.3g
Sugar: 3.5g
Fiber: 3.5g
Protein: 4.3g

Blend your leafy greens with water for 3 minutes and add your fruits and blend for another 2-3 minutes. Blend until your smoothie has a creamy consistency. We have come to the end of the first day. If you are feeling some symptoms such as nausea, cravings, headache, fatigue, pain and irritability, it is completely normal because your body is trying to adjust to the lack of solid food in your system. Embrace the changes and do not give up as it will get better the longer you stick with the program. Remember that you can snack in between meals in order to curb your appetite

DAY 2

If you want to, you can do some stretches and exercise for about 10-15 minutes just to get yourself ready for the day.

- [ ] **Breakfast Green Smoothie:** For your day 2 breakfast smoothie you will need:

- [ ] Protein powder
- [ ] 1 ripe or frozen banana
- [ ] 125ml of chopped pineapples
- [ ] 2 handfuls of spring mixed greens

- ☐ Water
- ☐ 2 handfuls of spinach
- ☐ ½ apple
- ☐ Almond milk

☐ **Nutritional Facts:**

Calories: 250kcal
Saturated Fat: 2g
Sugar: 39g
Fiber: 12g
Protein: 10g
Carbohydrates: 30g

Using a high powered blender, put your ingredients in the blender starting with the spring mixed greens and spinach and blend for 3-5 minutes until your smoothie has a creamy consistency.

☐ **Lunch green smoothie:** For this lunch green smoothie you will need:

- ☐ 2 handfuls of Kale
- ☐ Water
- ☐ Stevia as a sweetener
- ☐ 1 cup of coconut milk
- ☐ Grapes
- ☐ 1 medium fresh or frozen banana
- ☐ Berries (any type that you have)
- ☐ Greek yoghurt

☐ **Nutritional Facts:**

Calories: 320kcal
Carbohydrates: 40g
Total fats: 10g
Sugar: 42g
Fiber: 29g
Protein: 15g

Blend the ingredients in a blender and you can do it in stages so that you can get the consistency you want. Using Stevia, does not add any extra calories which makes it an excellent choice if you want your smoothie a little sweeter. If you feel hungry, you can try eating some healthy snacks and fruits to curb your hunger.

☐ **Dinner green smoothie:** For your dinner smoothie, you will need the following ingredients:

- ☐ Protein powder
- ☐ Berries (if you have more than one type, you can use both in your smoothie)
- ☐ 1 large handful of spinach or kale
- ☐ 2 cups of almond milk
- ☐ Chia seed
- ☐ Water

☐ Nutritional Facts:

Calories: 180kcal
Carbohydrates: 15g
Total fats: 5g
Sugar: 30g
Fiber: 2g
Protein: 12g

Place your ingredients in a high powered blender and blend until your smoothie has a creamy consistency. This brings us to the end of day two. Remember if you still feel that you are not ready to take smoothies three times a day, you can opt for a light salad. If you are feeling some of the symptoms of cleansing, try taking some pain killers or going to bed early.

DAY 3

It is your third day of your 12-day smoothie meal plan and you have to give yourself a pat on the back for making it through the first two challenging days. By now, you should be weaning yourself off eating light dinners and be ready to replace your dinner with a glass of green smoothie. If you have been taking green smoothies three times a day for the past two days, congratulate yourself and let's get into today's meal plan.

☐ Breakfast green smoothie:

- ☐ 1 cup of spinach
- ☐ ½ of an apple
- ☐ 1 cup of pineapples
- ☐ 2 ripe or frozen bananas
- ☐ Chia seeds
- ☐ Water

☐ Nutritional Facts:

Calories: 230kcal

Carbohydrates: 30g
Total fats: 7g
Sugar: 31g
Fiber: 8g
Protein: 3g

☐ **Lunch green smoothie:**

- ☐ Protein powder
- ☐ Chia seeds
- ☐ Unsweetened peanut butter
- ☐ 1 ripe or frozen banana
- ☐ 2 handfuls of spinach
- ☐ 1 handful of mixed berries

☐ **Nutritional Facts:**

Calories: 200kcal
Carbohydrates: 40g
Total fats: 20g
Sugar: 13g
Fiber: 2g
Protein: 26g

This takes 2 minutes to prepare and it will help you remain fuller for longer. If you feel it needs a little more flavor, you are free to add stevia in it to sweeten it.

☐ **Dinner green smoothie:**

- ☐ Coconut milk
- ☐ A handful or 2 of Kale
- ☐ Turmeric powder
- ☐ Protein powder (optional)
- ☐ Flax seeds
- ☐ Water
- ☐ A cup of pineapples

☐ **Nutritional Facts:**

Calories: 230kcal
Carbohydrates: 15g
Total fats: 18g
Sugar: 21g
Fiber: 2.9g
Protein: 32g

We have come to the end of the third day. If you need to take a snack go ahead but make sure it is a healthy one and you can also try eating some of the fruits you bought as snacks.

DAY 4

Welcome to the fourth day of your smoothie meal plan. By now, your body has started getting used to not having as many calories as it usually gets and is trying to maximize the little it is getting. If you wish to add exercise to your diet plan, do so but try to do nothing that will wear you out.

☐ **Breakfast green smoothie**

☐ 1 banana
☐ ½ of an apple
☐ 2 tablespoons of chia seeds
☐ 1-2 cups of water
☐ 1-2 cups of pineapple
☐ 2 cups of spinach or kale (use the one available)

☐ **Nutritional Facts:**

Calories: 250kcal
Carbohydrates: 25g
Total fats: 9g
Sugar: 21g
Fiber: 3.2g
Protein: 36g

☐ **Lunch green smoothie**

☐ Greek yoghurt
☐ Flax seeds
☐ 2 cups of Swiss chard
☐ 1 small handful of kale
☐ 2 cups of pineapple
☐ Grapes

☐ **Nutritional Facts:**

Calories: 200kcal
Carbohydrates: 30g
Total fats: 9g
Sugar: 11g
Fiber: 2.1g
Protein: 30g

- ☐ **Dinner green smoothie**

- ☐ Water
- ☐ Protein powder (optional)
- ☐ 2 handfuls of spinach
- ☐ Berries (either blueberries or strawberries)
- ☐ Chia seeds
- ☐ 1 handful of Swiss chard

- ☐ **Nutritional Facts:**

Calories: 140kcal
Carbohydrates: 11g
Total fats: 6g
Sugar: 5g
Fiber: 1.3g
Protein: 15g

We have come to the end of the fourth day of the 12-day green smoothie meal plan. For snacks, try eating some nuts and fruits.

DAY 5

- ☐ **Breakfast Green smoothie**

- ☐ 1 ripe or frozen banana
- ☐ A handful of spinach
- ☐ ¼ cup of avocado
- ☐ Protein based powder (optional)
- ☐ ½ cup of pineapple
- ☐ 1 tsp of chia seeds
- ☐ ½ cup of coconut milk

- ☐ **Nutritional Facts:**

Calories: 300kcal
Carbohydrates: 34g
Total fats: 23g
Sugar: 27g
Fiber: 4.5g
Protein: 32g

- ☐ **Lunch green smoothie**

- ☐ Greek yoghurt
- ☐ Flax seeds

- ☐ 2 handfuls of kale
- ☐ Grapes
- ☐ ½ of an apple
- ☐ Water

☐ **Nutritional Facts:**

Calories: 190kcal
Carbohydrates: 10g
Total fats: 8g
Sugar: 4g
Fiber: 3.1g
Protein: 21g

☐ **Dinner green smoothie**

- ☐ Protein based powder (optional)
- ☐ 1 handful of Swiss chard
- ☐ 1 cup of almond milk
- ☐ 1 tsp of chia seeds
- ☐ Water
- ☐ Berries
- ☐ 1 cup of frozen peaches

☐ **Nutritional Facts:**

Calories: 160kcal
Carbohydrates: 15g
Total fats: 8g
Sugar: 14g
Fiber: 2.3g
Protein: 11g

DAY 6

☐ **Breakfast green smoothie**

- ☐ Water
- ☐ 1-2 cups of frozen peaches
- ☐ 2 handfuls of kale
- ☐ 1 cup of pineapples
- ☐ Protein based powder (optional)
- ☐ Almond milk

☐ **Nutritional Facts:**

Calories: 240kcal

Carbohydrates: 20g
Total fats: 20g
Sugar: 18g
Fiber: 5.8g
Protein: 20g

☐ **Lunch green smoothie**

- ☐ Water
- ☐ I tsp of chia seeds
- ☐ Swiss chard
- ☐ Greek yoghurt
- ☐ ½ cup of apple
- ☐ 1 ripe or frozen banana

☐ **Nutritional Facts:**

Calories: 300kcal
Carbohydrates: 32g
Total fats: 25g
Sugar: 18g
Fiber: 5.9g
Protein: 29g

☐ **Dinner green smoothie**

- ☐ Water
- ☐ Protein powder (optional)
- ☐ 2 handfuls of spinach
- ☐ Berries (either blueberries or strawberries)
- ☐ Chia seeds
- ☐ 1 handful of Swiss chard

☐ **Nutritional Facts:**

Calories: 180kcal
Carbohydrates: 6g
Total fats: 4g
Sugar: 5g
Fiber: 1.5g
Protein: 7g

DAY 7

☐ **Breakfast green smoothie**

- ☐ Water

- ☐ 1-2 cups of frozen peaches
- ☐ 2 handfuls of kale
- ☐ 1 cup of pineapples
- ☐ Protein based powder (optional)
- ☐ Almond milk

☐ Nutritional Facts:

Calories: 200kcal
Carbohydrates: 22g
Total fats: 14g
Sugar: 4g
Fiber: 5g
Protein: 23g

☐ Lunch green smoothie

- ☐ 1 cup of coconut milk
- ☐ 1 tsp of turmeric powder
- ☐ 2 cups of spring mixed greens
- ☐ ½ cup if apple
- ☐ Grapes

☐ Nutritional Facts:

Calories: 190kcal
Carbohydrates: 8g
Total fats: 15g
Sugar: 10g
Fiber: 2g
Protein: 27g

☐ Dinner green smoothie

- ☐ Berries
- ☐ Water
- ☐ Protein based powder (optional)
- ☐ 2 handfuls of spinach
- ☐ 1 cup of almond milk

☐ Nutritional Facts:

Calories: 130kcal
Carbohydrates: 10g
Total fats: 6g
Sugar: 4g
Fiber: 2.8g

Protein: 19g

WEEK TWO

Congratulations on finishing the first week. Since the shopping list provided was for the first week alone, here is what you are going to need for the second week:

- Bananas
- Apples
- Unsalted nuts to snack on
- Spinach
- Avocado
- Protein based powder (optional)
- Chia seeds
- Coconut milk
- Pomegranates
- Frozen mangoes
- Mixed berries
- Pineapples
- Kale
- Spring mixed greens
- Fruits and veggies for you to snack on
- Flax seeds
- Almond milk
- Unsweetened peanut butter
- Greek yoghurt

After shopping, it is time to complete the remaining 5 days of your 12-day smoothie meal plan

DAY 8

☐ **Breakfast green smoothie**

☐ 1 ripe or frozen banana
☐ A handful of spinach
☐ ¼ cup of avocado
☐ Protein based powder (optional)
☐ ½ cup of pineapple
☐ 1 tsp of chia seeds
☐ ½ cup of coconut milk

☐ **Nutritional Facts:**

Calories: 220kcal

Carbohydrates: 14g
Total fats: 13g
Sugar: 6g
Fiber: 4.4g
Protein: 30g

☐ **Lunch green smoothie**

- ☐ Protein based powder (optional)
- ☐ Chia seeds
- ☐ Unsweetened peanut butter
- ☐ 1 ripe or frozen banana
- ☐ 2 handfuls of spinach
- ☐ 1 handful of mixed berries

☐ **Nutritional Facts:**

Calories: 240kcal
Carbohydrates: 45g
Total fats: 20g
Sugar: 13g
Fiber: 2g
Protein: 26g

☐ **Dinner green smoothie**

- ☐ 2 handfuls of kale
- ☐ 1 cup of mixed berries
- ☐ 1 cup of pomegranates
- ☐ ½ cup of apple
- ☐ Water
- ☐ Chia seeds
- ☐ 1 frozen banana

☐ **Nutritional Facts:**

Calories: 170kcal
Carbohydrates: 11g
Total fats: 5g
Sugar: 13g
Fiber: 4.4g
Protein: 16g

DAY 9

☐ **Breakfast green smoothie**

- ☐ 1 cup of coconut milk
- ☐ Chunks of frozen mangoes
- ☐ 2 handfuls of spring mixed greens
- ☐ Protein based powder (optional)
- ☐ 1 frozen or ripe banana
- ☐ Water
- ☐ 1 tsp of flax seeds

☐ **Nutritional Facts:**

Calories: 250kcal
Carbohydrates: 33g
Total fats: 17g
Sugar: 14g
Fiber: 2.7g
Protein: 36g

☐ **Lunch green smoothie**

- ☐ Greek yoghurt
- ☐ 1-2 large handfuls of spinach
- ☐ ½ cup of apple
- ☐ 1 cup of pineapples
- ☐ ½ cup of frozen mangoes

☐ **Nutritional Facts:**

Calories: 150kcal
Carbohydrates: 40g
Total fats: 4g
Sugar: 9g
Fiber: 5.2g
Protein: 17g

☐ **Dinner green smoothie**

- ☐ 1 cup of almond milk
- ☐ 1 cup of mixed berries
- ☐ 1 tsp of chia seeds
- ☐ 1 cup of pomegranates
- ☐ Protein based powder (optional)
- ☐ 2 handfuls of kale
- ☐ Water

☐ **Nutritional Facts:**

Calories: 202kcal

Carbohydrates: 23g
Total fats: 9g
Sugar: 13g
Fiber: 6g
Protein: 28g

DAY 10

☐ Breakfast green smoothie

- ☐ 1 cup of pomegranates
- ☐ 2 large handfuls of spinach
- ☐ ½ cup of avocado
- ☐ 1 cup of almond milk
- ☐ Water
- ☐ ½ cup of frozen mangoes
- ☐ Protein based powder (optional)

☐ Nutritional Facts:

Calories: 170kcal
Carbohydrates: 10g
Total fats: 17g
Sugar: 18g
Fiber: 12g
Protein: 29g

☐ Lunch green smoothie

- ☐ Protein based powder (optional)
- ☐ Chia seeds
- ☐ Unsweetened peanut butter
- ☐ 1 ripe or frozen banana
- ☐ 2 handfuls of spinach
- ☐ Water
- ☐ 1 handful of mixed berries

☐ Nutritional Facts:

Calories: 260kcal
Carbohydrates: 36g
Total fats: 14g
Sugar: 7.5g
Fiber: 11g
Protein: 18g

☐ Dinner green smoothie

- ☐ Water
- ☐ 1-2 cups of frozen peaches
- ☐ 2 handfuls of kale
- ☐ 1 cup of pineapples
- ☐ 1 cup of pomegranates
- ☐ Protein based powder (optional)
- ☐ Almond milk

☐ Nutritional Facts:

Calories: 150kcal
Carbohydrates: 40g
Total fats: 15g
Sugar: 18g
Fiber: 7.9g
Protein: 34g

DAY 11

☐ **Breakfast green smoothie**

- ☐ 2 handfuls of spring mixed greens
- ☐ 1 cup of frozen peaches
- ☐ 1 ripe or frozen banana
- ☐ 1 cup of almond milk
- ☐ ½ cup of pomegranates
- ☐ Water
- ☐ ½ cup of apples

☐ **Nutritional Facts:**

Calories: 225kcal
Carbohydrates: 14g
Total fats: 5.45g
Sugar: 10g
Fiber: 2g
Protein: 23g

☐ **Lunch green smoothie**

- ☐ Water
- ☐ I tsp of chia seeds
- ☐ 2 handfuls of kale
- ☐ Greek yoghurt
- ☐ ½ cup of apple

- ☐ 1 ripe or frozen banana

☐ **Nutritional Facts:**

Calories: 182.2kcal
Carbohydrates: 4g
Total fats: 10.5g
Sugar: 8g
Fiber: 8g
Protein: 25g

☐ **Dinner green smoothie**

- ☐ 1 cup of coconut milk
- ☐ 1 cup of frozen mangoes
- ☐ 1 tsp of flax seeds
- ☐ 1 cup of pomegranates
- ☐ Water
- ☐ ½ cup of avocado

☐ **Nutritional Facts:**

Calories: 205kcal
Carbohydrates: 16g
Total fats: 26g
Sugar: 18g
Fiber: 13g
Protein: 23g

DAY 12

We have come to the final day of this diet, be proud of yourself for sticking with it and seeing it through because not everyone can do what you did. Let's see what the final day holds.

☐ **Breakfast green smoothie**

- ☐ Protein based powder (optional)
- ☐ 2 large handfuls of kale
- ☐ 1 cup of mixed berries
- ☐ 1 tsp of chia seeds
- ☐ 1 cup of almond milk
- ☐ 1 cup of pineapples

☐ **Nutritional Facts:**

Calories: 195kcal

Carbohydrates: 31g
Total fats: 19g
Sugar: 16g
Fiber: 10g
Protein: 21g

☐ Lunch green smoothie

- ☐ Greek yoghurt
- ☐ 1 cup of pomegranates
- ☐ 1 cup of mixed berries
- ☐ 2 handfuls of spring mixed greens
- ☐ 1 frozen or fresh banana
- ☐ Protein based powder (optional)
- ☐ Water
- ☐ ½ a cup of apples

☐ Nutritional Facts:

Calories: 150kcal
Carbohydrates: 6g
Total fats: 5.2g
Sugar: 14g
Fiber: 6.3g
Protein: 23g

☐ Dinner green smoothie

- ☐ 1 banana
- ☐ ½ of an apple
- ☐ 1 cup of frozen mangoes
- ☐ 1 cup of water
- ☐ 1 cup of pineapple
- ☐ 2 handfuls of spinach or kale
- ☐ 1 cup of almond milk

☐ Nutritional Facts:

Calories: 195kcal
Carbohydrates: 15g
Total fats: 20g
Sugar: 10.1g
Fiber: 4.1g
Protein: 16g

We are officially done with the 12-day green smoothie plan, and all the weight you wanted to lose should be gone by now. Do not jump right into solid foods and make sure you take light foods first and make green smoothie a part of your everyday meal plan.

Things To Note While On a Diet

- **Add protein to your smoothie.** Adding protein to your smoothie is optional as it can make your smoothie taste "weird," but an extra scoop of protein in your smoothie will keep you feeling full for a while. Since you are avoiding dairy-based products in this diet, make sure the protein powder you wish to use is a non-dairy based protein powder. Try taking your smoothie with a protein-based powder to figure out if it works for you, and if it does not, you can leave it out.

- **There are certain extra ingredients you can use to spice things up.** If you want your green smoothie to have a little extra flavor, you can try adding turmeric, cinnamon, mint, ginger, parsley, basil, and ground red pepper to spice up your smoothie.

- **Keep your bowels moving.** One of the 12-day green smoothie diet's aims is to clear your body of the toxins, preventing it from functioning properly; therefore, your bowels must move at least 1-3 times a day. If you haven't moved your bowels in 24 hours, try drinking Celtic sea salt with water. If you cannot tolerate the taste of the sea salt, you can add fresh lemon juice to it.

- **Make sure you drink herbal teas.** While coffee is not allowed during this cleanse, there is nothing wrong with you drinking herbal tea once in a while. In fact, drinking herbal tea will contribute positively to your losing weight during the cleanse. Herbal teas like green tea, peppermint, chamomile, ginger, ginseng, and dandelion root, are good teas that you can drink to aid the detoxification process.

- **Do not eat the same greens.** As much as possible, try to rotate the greens you consume in order to avoid a toxic build up in your system. If you used spinach this week, try using kale the next week and mixed greens afterward. You could also use different types of greens during the week and switch it up the next week. Apart from spinach, kale, Swiss chard, and mixed greens used in the 12-day green smoothie meal plan, other leafy greens that you can use include dandelion greens and mustard greens, arugula turnip greens, etc.

- **Avoid starving yourself.** As much as you want to lose weight, this meal plan does not support starvation. Have a healthy snack in between smoothies when you feel hungry. Also, make sure you drink a lot of water while on this diet as it helps in the detoxification process.

- **Expect cleansing symptoms.** When you start experiencing symptoms such as headache, nausea, cravings, fatigue, pains, irritability, rashes, and muscle ache, it is not a sign that you should give up the diet but that you are doing something right. As you stick with the diet, the symptoms eventually go away, leaving you feeling refreshed and lighter since your body has gotten rid of most of the toxins in your system. If you cannot bear the symptoms, try taking a painkiller and resting a little until you feel better.

- **De-stem your vegetables.** Many of the packaged vegetables do not have stems any more, but to be on the safe side, make sure to check if their stems had been removed before putting them in the blender.

You can use either ripe fruits or frozen fruits. Using ripe fruits in your green smoothie makes it easier to digest because of its live enzymes. If the fruits you have are not ripe, allow it to ripen for a while before using it. Most people prefer using frozen fruits because it gives the green smoothie an almost ice-cream-like texture, and if you want to use it instead of ripe fruits, go ahead. The nutritional value of frozen fruits is the same as fresh fruits; plus, it would take longer for them to spoil. While you can use most fruits in their frozen form, it is advisable that you use the apples and bananas fresh.

There is no reason for your green smoothie to taste bad. Just because you are using vegetables in it does not mean that your smoothie has to taste nasty. As you continue on in the diet, you can modify it to suit your needs. You can also use sweeteners preferably Stevia to sweeten it. You can also replace water with almond milk. After the diet, there is no harm with trying to come up with recipes of your own to suit your needs.

CHAPTER 3

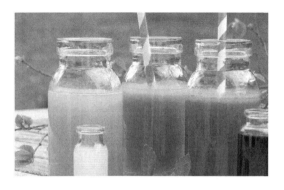

MORE GREEN SMOOTHIE RECIPES

After the diet, it is important that you take green smoothies at least once to twice a day, but having one style of making green smoothies can be very boring. Luckily for us, there are a lot of other ways you can make your green smoothies and other ingredients that you can try to give it another taste and edge. Now that you are done with the diet, here are other ways to make your green smoothie and ingredients that you can use.

☐ **Green and Peaches**
For this smoothie you will need:

☐ 1 cup of strawberries (preferably frozen)
☐ 2 cups of water
☐ 1 cup of peaches (preferably frozen)
☐ 1 tablespoon of flax seeds (grounded)
☐ 1 packet of Stevia
☐ 2 handfuls of Spinach
☐ 1 small handful of Kale

Using a high powered blender, place your ingredients starting with the leafy greens and water and blend slowly. If you are using a regular blender, try separating the ingredients into two parts to avoid chunky vegetables. Blend for at least 4-5 minutes or until your smoothie has a creamy smooth consistency.

☐ **Going Basic**
For this smoothie you will need:

☐ 1-2 cups of mixed fruits or mixed berries
☐ 1 cup of soy milk or almond milk
☐ 2 handfuls of arugula

- ☐ ½ cup of water
- ☐ 1 tablespoon of flax seeds

Place all ingredients in a blender and blend slowly until it has a smooth and creamy consistency. Start with the leafy greens and milk if you want your smoothie to have a little bit of thickness and blend for at least 5 minutes.

☐ **Time to Glow**
For this smoothie you will need:

- ☐ 2 large handfuls of spinach
- ☐ ½ a cup of avocado
- ☐ 2 cups of almond milk
- ☐ 1 ½ cups of frozen chunks of mangoes or pineapples (preferably pineapples)
- ☐ Stevia (if you need extra sweetness)
- ☐ 1 tablespoon of chia seeds

Place your ingredients in a blender and blend for 3-5 minutes or until your smoothie is smooth and has a creamy consistency. Add a little more almond milk if you like it thicker and add a packet of stevia if you need the additional sweetness.

☐ **Berries Splash**
For this smoothie you will need:

- ☐ 2 cups of mixed berries
- ☐ 1 apple
- ☐ 2 handfuls of spinach
- ☐ A small handful of spring mixed greens
- ☐ 1 cup of water
- ☐ 1 cup of unsweetened Greek yoghurt
- ☐ 1 tablespoon of flax seeds.

Start with the greens, a little bit of water and Greek yoghurt and blend slowly for 2 minutes. Add the remaining ingredients and blend for an additional 3 minutes or until your smoothie is to your liking.

☐ **Peachy berries**
For this smoothie you will need:

- ☐ 2 cups of frozen peaches
- ☐ 1 apple
- ☐ 1 ½ cups of mixed berries
- ☐ 1 tsp of vanilla
- ☐ 2 large handfuls of spring mixed greens or arugula

- ☐ I handful of spinach
- ☐ Water

Put your ingredients in a blender starting with the greens and water and blend until your smoothie has a smooth and creamy consistency.

☐ Turmeric Mango
For this smoothie you will need:

- ☐ 2 cups of frozen or fresh mangoes (preferably fresh)
- ☐ 2 cups of kale or spinach
- ☐ 1 tablespoon of turmeric
- ☐ Water
- ☐ ½ cup of apple

Place all of your ingredients in a blender and blend until it is smooth. You can add toppings if you want.

☐ Tropical Turmeric
For this smoothie you will need:

- ☐ ¼ cup of lemon juice (fresh)
- ☐ 1 cup of pineapple1 tablespoon of turmeric
- ☐ 1 tsp of ginger
- ☐ 2 handfuls of Kale
- ☐ 1 cup of coconut milk
- ☐ Water if necessary

Start with your greens and coconut milk and blend slowly for 2 minutes. Add the remaining ingredients and blend until it is smooth.

☐ Burn it away
For this smoothie you will need:

- ☐ ½ a cup of coconut milk
- ☐ ½ a cup of avocado
- ☐ Water
- ☐ Lemon juice
- ☐ 2 cups of green tea
- ☐ 2 handfuls of spinach

Blend for at least 5 minutes or until it is smooth and has a creamy consistency. You can add protein based powder if you want.

☐ Chocolate green smoothie
For this smoothie you will need:

- [ ] 2-3 tablespoons of cacao powder
- [ ] 2 handfuls of spring mixed greens or spinach
- [ ] 1 cup of water
- [ ] 1 cup of Greek yoghurt
- [ ] 1 cup of cherries
- [ ] 1 large frozen banana

Place your ingredients in a blender starting with the leafy greens and blend for at least 5 minutes.

- [ ] **Coconut Mango Bliss**
For this smoothie you will need:

- [ ] 1 cup of coconut milk or coconut water
- [ ] 1 cup of water
- [ ] 2 cups of kale
- [ ] 1 cup of frozen chunks of mangoes
- [ ] Stevia to sweeten
- [ ] 1 tablespoon of protein powder

Place your ingredients in a blender and blend slowly for 5 minutes. If you need your smoothie a little thicker, you can add more coconut milk. Use the stevia if you need your smoothie a little sweeter.

CHAPTER 4

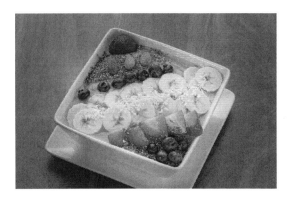

HEALTHY SNACKING AND EXERCISING

Anytime you are on a diet or just trying to maintain your weight, I am sure that your nutritionist must have kept reminding you to eat more often and eat a snack or two but instead of you to ask him/her what they really mean when they tell you to eat snacks, you take it as permission for you to indulge yourself in anything you like especially unhealthy snacks. As I mentioned in the first chapter, it is completely okay for you to indulge in some healthy snacks once in a while, and if you feel like you are up to it, you can also try exercising but ensure you do nothing that will stress you out and make you hungry. But what after your diet? How can you keep up with the healthy snacks and exercising, especially when you have no zeal or interest to do both? When people hear the word "snack," they immediately think about ice cream, Oreos, M&Ms, cookies, chips, and other high calorie processed foods, but that is not what snacking is about. Snacking means eating or drinking something in between meals, whether it is healthy or not. Research has shown that a lot of people choose to snack even when eaten or are about to eat, and when asked why they would choose to eat unhealthy snacks, most of them simply said that they ate it as a result of temptation because they were hungry. Whether the snacks you decide to eat are healthy or not, it is not a hidden secret that snacking has a huge impact on your health and can help influence your weight loss or weight gain as the case may be. Some people argue that when you break down your food intake in a day into small meals and snacks, it will help to reduce your calorie intake compared to when you eat three huge meals a day because snacking every few hours would help to boost your metabolism. However, there is no scientific evidence backing it up. In fact, research has shown that whether a person eats three huge high carb meals a day or seven little ones, the calorie intake remains the same (if the meals are eaten are the same).

EFFECT OF SNACKING ON APPETITE

For nutritionists and scientists alike, the question of whether snacking has a significant influence on weight gain is still a highly debated issue. We all know that snacking can help to reduce hunger and keep you feeling satisfied for a while, especially on those days where your meals are set hours apart from each other. When it comes to the effect of snacking on appetite, there is no universally agreed-upon conclusion because all studies that have been conducted on people with different body types come out with different results. Some results showed that for some individuals, snacking between meals and late at night, does not make any difference in their total calorie intake or in their hunger levels compared to the days they ate no snacks at all. At the same time, studies have also shown that snacking has helped to curb appetite and hunger. In a study conducted with women with obesity, it was noted that a snack that was high in protein or carbs, led to the women feeling less hungry in the morning. So, the effects of snacking on a person largely depend on the type of snack that is being consumed and the individual's make-up. Whether you are losing weight or just trying to maintain it, snacking is something that you cannot avoid, and for you not to sabotage your weight loss efforts, try to reach out to a nutritionist so that you can find out what works best for you.

EFFECTS OF SNACKING ON WEIGHT GAIN AND LOSS

Like the results of snacking on appetite, there are also varying opinions on the effects of snacking on weight gain and loss. Most researches have shown that snacking between meals does not affect a person's weight, depending on the type of snack eaten. When the snacks you eat are rich in protein with high fiber content, you might find yourself losing weight rather than gaining it. Still, the effects snacking has on the body with regards to weight still depends on the individual. A study conducted with obese people showed that snacking reduces the rate at which their body burns fat and can result in weight gain if the person is not careful. Apart from the individual, the effect of snacking on weight is also affected by the timing. For instance, if you eat a high-calorie snack late at night, you might not burn as much fat as you would like compared to when you ate such a snack in the afternoon or early evening. Our bodies react in different ways, and the best thing you can do for yourself is to understand what is best for your body and your health. Snacking as a part of your lifestyle is unavoidable, and as much as having a cheeseburger can be a burst of happiness at times, you need to know when to indulge yourself and when to hold yourself back from giving in to your cravings.

If you need ideas for healthy snacks you can eat between meals and for those late nights, here are some that you can try:

- **Peanut butter on apple:** Surprisingly, apples and peanut butter taste great together, and if you have not tried it before, you do not know what you are missing. When you are choosing the peanut butter to use on your apple, go for the natural unsweetened one. Peanut butter is still fairly high in calories so, ensure that you use it in moderation.

- **Honey-cinnamon water:** There is no reason for you to drink plain water if you want to lose weight as this honey and cinnamon combo can do the job for you. Cinnamon has been proven to speed up the metabolic rate for weight loss, so when you combine it with honey and warm water, you will find yourself losing weight while you sleep and during the day.

- **Cottage cheese with avocado:** Cottage cheese has very few calories because it is filled with natural proteins that instantly make you feel full. Avocados are good sources of healthy fat, and combining it with cottage cheese will not only help you lose weight or maintain your weight but would also help reduce your cholesterol levels and aid your cardiovascular system.

- **Mixed nuts:** Nuts are nutritious snacks because they provide a balance of healthy fat, fiber, and protein. They are low in calories, do not need refrigeration as they do not spoil easily, and you can just throw them in your bed and snack on them throughout the day. Plus, studies have also shown that eating nuts moderately, can aid your weight loss.

- **Guacamoles with red bell peppers:** Guacamoles are dips made from avocados and are considered to be very healthy so, when you pair them with red bell peppers that are also packed with nutrients and antioxidants, you will find that you do not need to each much of it for you to be satisfied and the best part is together, they are low in calories and would not adversely affect your calorie intake.

- **Pineapple juice:** If you are not on a diet but still want to keep the belly fat away, drinking pineapple juice is one of the best decisions you can make. Pineapple juice contains an enzyme called bromelain, which metabolizes protein and helps to burn excess belly fat.

- **Greek yogurt with berries:** When looking for foods that help to lose or maintain weight, Greek yogurt is always listed as one of the best options. Greek yogurt is high in protein, which helps you to feel full without you eating much, and berries are an excellent source of antioxidants. Combining berries with Greek yogurt will not only help you lose weight but would also provide your body with lots of nutrients and antioxidants.

- **Cinnamon with cottage cheese and flax seeds:** Not only will it aid in your weight loss, but it would also help you to control your blood sugar and improve your gut health.

- **Carrot sticks with hummus dips:** This is an ideal night snack as it would make you feel full as it is rich in fiber, fatty acids, and high-quality proteins. The hummus dip is relatively easy to make, and since you can find carrots anywhere, it is a snack that you can have in your home and by your bedside all the time.

- **Dark Chocolate:** Dark chocolate is a rich and satisfying snack, which makes it an excellent choice when on a diet. Besides helping to keep you satisfied, dark chocolate also helps to reduce the risk of heart disease and can help lower blood pressure.

- **Chickpeas:** Chickpeas have a nutty texture and meaty flavor with a high fiber content that is good for your body. Plus, it is something that you can carry around with you and snack on throughout the day.

- **Grapes, oranges, pears, and other fruits:** When it seems like there is no creative snack idea left to try, you can always fall back on fruits and eating fruits, which can be very satisfying.

- **Hard-boiled eggs:** Eggs are one of the healthiest snacks you can eat while on a diet. Eggs are very filling and can help you reduce the number of calories you eat in a day, which would, in turn, lead to weight loss. Although they are also known for their high cholesterol content, studies have shown that consuming eggs in moderation does not increase the risk of heart disease.

EXERCISING

Having excess weight is not fun. Not only does it make you sluggish and tired easily, but it is also the leading cause of a majority of diseases. Many diets out there serve as a rapid-fire way to burn fat, but the oldest and most trustworthy way to burn that unwanted fat will always be exercise. Some people rely on exercise alone to get the body of their dreams while others are making the best of both worlds by combining exercising with their preferred diet to achieve quick and impressive results. Exercise alone without a proper diet and nutrition plan is a pure waste of time because the only thing you do is to burn the fat only to add it back with the food you eat. What do you stand to gain by combining exercise with the right diet?

Most people depend on calorie restriction to help them lose excess weight; however, combining exercise with a healthy diet seems to be more effective than that. When you combine exercise with a healthy diet, you are preventing your body from being affected by certain diseases since you are giving your body the nutrients that it needs as well as building it up. You help prevent your body from health conditions like high blood pressure, high cholesterol levels, and cancer when you exercise. Not only will exercising build you up physically, but it would also build you up mentally and increase your confidence and self-esteem. Exercising at first is never easier, but when you resist the temptation to quit and keep doing it day in and day out, you will feel pleased with yourself for sticking to something and seeing it through even on the days when you do not want to get up from your bed. By building your confidence and self-esteem, exercise helps to relieve a person of their anxiety or depression or at least lower it.

Exercise is instrumental in losing weight and keeping the weight off. During your 12-day smoothie diet, doing exercises on some days will help speed up your weight loss process. Even after the diet, it is still important for you to exercise once in a while so that the weight you lost would not come back. Exercise helps to increase metabolism, which allows your body to burn more calories than it initially would plus, it helps to maintain and build muscle and lean body mass, which also helps to increase how many calories you burn in a day. Combining exercise with your diet would also help you feel and look youthful. From your diet, your body gets all sorts of antioxidants and nutrients which it uses to maintain itself and fight the aging process, and exercising can prevent your body from feeling the effects of aging such as soreness and stiffness since you are moving around as much as you can. Since your body is loaded with all the nutrients it needs, exercising helps your body not only to maintain itself but also to build a strong immune system capable of handling germs and maintaining the body's functions. A poor diet with no exercise and lots of sugar and processed foods can stop your body from getting the amount of sleep that it needs, which can compromise your body's health. Without getting enough sleep, you might not be able to function on your own throughout the day without the aid of coffee. Those that are physically active and maintain a proper diet are able to sleep better at night and feel good about themselves when they wake up in the morning.

With all the benefits exercising provides, how much exercise does the body need to lose weight? Some spend at least one to two hours a day doing vigorous exercises to stay fit and lose weight, however, since you are on a diet, the goal is to do as much exercise as you can without stressing yourself out. Doing 20 minutes of aerobic exercises or 15 minutes of walking three times a week, combined with your diet, can help you burn up more calories and keep your body burning calories even at night. Since your body is already trying to maximize the few calories that it is getting, it is recommended that you do not try to do any high-intensity workout that will leave you breathless in seconds as it would do your body no good. Stick to cardio, yoga, or simple stretches if you wish to include exercising in your 12-day green smoothie meal plan. After your diet plan has been done, you can increase the amount of time you work out daily and try to incorporate some high-intensity workouts in it as well. Each day, try to focus on a different part of your body in order to get a toned physique. As I have mentioned earlier, going through the 12-day green smoothie diet is one thing, but maintaining your weight and not falling back to your old routine is an entirely new ballgame. By sticking to a healthy diet and exercise, you will not only maintain your weight, but your body will thank you in the long run.

CHAPTER 5

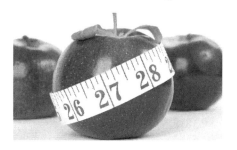

TRACK YOUR PROGRESS AND SEE RESULTS

	BREAKFAST	LUNCH	DINNER
WEEK ONE GREEN SMOOTHIE MEAL PLAN			
MONDAY	Water Protein powder (optional) 2 handfuls of spinach Berries Chia seeds 1 handful of Swiss chard	6oz of Greek yoghurt Coconut milk 1 ripe or frozen banana 2-4 cups of Spinach or Kale Water	Water Protein powder (optional) 2 handfuls of spinach Berries Chia seeds 1 handful of Swiss chard
TUESDAY	Protein powder 1 ripe or frozen banana 125ml of chopped pineapples 2 handfuls of spring mixed greens Water 2 handfuls of spinach ½ apple Almond milk	2 handfuls of Kale Water Stevia as a sweetener 1 cup of coconut milk Grapes 1 medium fresh or frozen banana Berries Greek yoghurt	Protein powder Berries 1 large handful of spinach or kale 2 cups of almond milk Chia seed Water
WEDNESDAY	1cup of spinach	Protein powder	Coconut milk

	½ of an apple 1 cup of pineapples 2 ripe or frozen bananas Chia seeds Water	Chia seeds 1 ripe or frozen banana 2 handfuls of spinach 1 handful of mixed berries	A handful or 2 of Kale Turmeric powder Protein powder Flax seeds Water A cup of pineapples
THURSDAY	1 banana ½ of an apple 2 tablespoons of chia seeds 1-2 cups of water 1-2 cups of pineapple 2 cups of spinach or kale (use the one available)	Greek yoghurt Flax seeds 2 cups of Swiss chard 1 small handful of kale 2 cups of pineapple Grapes	Water Protein powder (optional) 2 handfuls of spinach Berries Chia seeds 1 handful of Swiss chard
FRIDAY	1 ripe or frozen banana A handful of spinach ¼ cup of avocado Protein based powder (optional) ½ cup of pineapple 1 tsp of chia seeds ½ cup of coconut milk	Greek yoghurt Flax seeds 2 handfuls of kale Grapes ½ of an apple Water	Protein based powder (optional) 1 handful of Swiss chard 1 cup of almond milk 1 tsp of chia seeds Water Berries 1 cup of frozen peaches
SATURDAY	Water 1-2 cups of frozen peaches 2 handfuls of kale 1 cup of pineapples Protein based	Water I tsp of chia seeds Swiss chard Greek yoghurt ½ cup of apple 1 ripe or frozen banana	Water Protein powder (optional) 2 handfuls of spinach Berries Chia seeds 1 handful of Swiss chard

	powder (optional) Almond milk		
SUNDAY	Water 1-2 cups of frozen peaches 2 handfuls of kale 1 cup of pineapples Protein based powder (optional) Almond milk	1 cup of coconut milk 1 tsp of turmeric powder 2 cups of spring mixed greens ½ cup if apple Grapes	Berries Water Protein based powder (optional) 2 handfuls of spinach 1 cup of almond milk

WEEK TWO OF GREEN SMOOTHIE DIET

	BREAKFAST	LUNCH	DINNER
MONDAY	1 ripe or frozen banana A handful of spinach ¼ cup of avocado Protein based powder (optional) ½ cup of pineapple 1 tsp of chia seeds ½ cup of coconut milk	Protein based powder (optional) Chia seeds Unsweetened peanut butter 1 ripe or frozen banana 2 handfuls of spinach 1 handful of mixed berries	2 handfuls of kale 1 cup of mixed berries 1 cup of pomegranates ½ cup of apple Water Chia seeds 1 frozen banana
TUESDAY	1 cup of coconut milk Chunks of frozen mangoes 2 handfuls of spring mixed greens Protein based powder	Greek yoghurt 1-2 large handfuls of spinach ½ cup of apple 1 cup of pineapples ½ cup of frozen	1 cup of almond milk 1 cup of mixed berries 1 tsp of chia seeds 1 cup of pomegranates Protein based powder (optional) 2 handfuls of kale Water

	(optional) 1 frozen or ripe banana Water 1 tsp of flax seeds	mangoes	
WEDNESDAY	1 cup of pomegranates 2 large handfuls of spinach ½ cup of avocado 1 cup of almond milk Water ½ cup of frozen mangoes Protein based powder (optional)	Protein based powder (optional) Chia seeds Unsweetened peanut butter 1 ripe or frozen banana 2 handfuls of spinach Water 1 handful of mixed berries	Water 1-2 cups of frozen peaches 2 handfuls of kale 1 cup of pineapples 1 cup of pomegranates Protein based powder (optional) Almond milk
THURSDAY	2 handfuls of spring mixed greens 1 cup of frozen peaches 1 ripe or frozen banana 1 cup of almond milk ½ cup of pomegranates Water ½ cup of apples	Water I tsp of chia seeds 2 handfuls of kale Greek yoghurt ½ cup of apple 1 ripe or frozen banana	1 cup of coconut milk 1 cup of frozen mangoes 1 tsp of flax seeds 1 cup of pomegranates Water ½ cup of avocado
FRIDAY	Protein based powder (optional) 2 large handfuls of kale 1 cup of mixed berries	Greek yoghurt 1 cup of pomegranates 1 cup of mixed berries 2 handfuls of spring mixed greens	1 banana ½ of an apple 1 cup of frozen mangoes 1 cup of water 1 cup of pineapple 2 handfuls of spinach or kale 1 cup of almond milk

	1 tsp of chia seeds 1 cup of almond milk 1 cup of pineapples	1 frozen or fresh banana Protein based powder (optional) Water ½ a cup of apples	
SATURDAY			
SUNDAY	DON'T	STOP	CONTINUE!

CONTINUE THE PLAN AFTER THE 12 DAYS!

TRACK YOUR MEALS DAILY

WEEKLY SMOOTHIE MEAL PLANNER

	BREAKFAST	LUNCH	DINNER
MONDAY			
TUESDAY			
WEDNESDAY			
THURSDAY			
FRIDAY			
SATURDAY			
SUNDAY			

WEEKLY SMOOTHIE MEAL PLANNER

	BREAKFAST	LUNCH	DINNER
MONDAY			
TUESDAY			
WEDNESDAY			
THURSDAY			
FRIDAY			
SATURDAY			
SUNDAY			

COMPLETE SHOPPING LIST FOR 2 WEEKS

- Apples
- Grapes
- Frozen Peaches
- Bananas
- Spinach
- Swiss Chard
- Water
- Pear
- Avocados
- Pineapples
- Chia seeds
- Flax seeds
- Turmeric powder
- Kale
- Stevia (to sweeten)
- Berries of different kinds like blueberries, strawberries etc.
- Spring mix greens
- Unsweetened peanut butter and nuts to snack on
- Greek yoghurt
- Almond milk
- Protein based powder (optional)
- Coconut milk
- Pomegranates
- Frozen mangoes
- Mixed berries
- Fruits and veggies for you to snack on

CONCLUSION

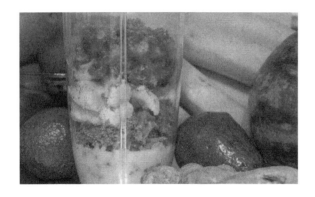

We have come to the end of the book, and I must congratulate you on finishing the book and the diet because not everyone can do that. It takes a lot of self-discipline and motivation, especially if you are a newbie, to stick to a diet plan that you had not done before. As I have said throughout this book, losing weight is one thing, but keeping the weight off is completely different. If you are not sure of the next step you should take after following this diet, try reaching out to a nutritionist so that you can have an idea of what is best for you. You could also try talking with other people that have been through this experience and find out what they do to remain in shape and how their green smoothie diet was for them. Also, try to eat balanced meals and avoid eating empty calories as much as you can. Try to eat foods rich in vitamins, fatty acids, proteins, minerals, and fiber as they will help your body function properly and maintain a healthy weight. Avoid sugar and salt because they do not have any nutritional value, and they are bad for your health; they also lead to bloating, water retention, and swelling. If you must eat red meat, limit it to two times a week or at most three. Instead of red meat, you can eat more chicken, turkey, brown rice, eggs, nuts, and other foods that are sources of good healthy fat. Eat more fresh and organic foods as they do not contain any chemical preservatives, antibiotics, additives, and hormones like packaged and frozen food. Also, fresh organic foods are less toxic than packaged foods. If you are trying to make a switch from coffee, try drinking green tea. The caffeine in green tea works differently from coffee as it improves your health, vitality, and stamina while leaving out the side effects of coffee. Being fit is an everyday commitment meaning that you must be willing to get up each morning and push yourself even when you do not want to. There is no rule against not having cheat days, but try to make sure that you are still eating healthy and putting your health and your body first. I am sure that this book has been a huge help to you

n your weight loss journey, and I hope you enjoyed reading the book
s much as I enjoyed writing it.

THANK YOU

Thank you for buying my book and I hope you enjoyed it. If you found any value in this book I would really appreciate it if you'd take a minute to post a review on Amazon about this book. I check all my reviews and love to get feedback.

This is the real reward for me knowing that I'm helping others. If you know anyone who may enjoy this book, please share the message and gift it to them.

As you work towards your goals, you may have questions or run into some issues. I'd like to be able to help you, so let's connect.

I don't charge for the assistance, so feel free to connect with me on the internet at:

Join the Smoothie Diet Lifestyle Change Facebook Group:

https://www.facebook.com/groups/2823120257784670/

Add Me As A Friend On Facebook:

https://www.facebook.com/Quinones-Stephanie-113966356909921/

ABOUT AUTHOR

My name is Stephanie Quiñones, an entrepreneur living in the United States who loves sharing knowledge and helping others on the topic of weight-loss, healthy eating, anti-aging, and improving love life.

I'm a very passionate person who will go the extra mile and over-delivers to inspire others to lose weight, be healthy, and to achieve the sexy body they desire.

Stephanie's words of wisdom:

"I believe that knowledge is power. Everyone should improve themselves and/or business, no matter what stage in life they're in. Whether it's to develop a better mindset or to increase profits. Moving forward is key."

Printed in Great Britain
by Amazon